Permanently Beat PCOS: The Complete Solution

Proven Step-by-Step Polycystic Ovarian Syndrome Guide to Improved Fertility, Weight Loss and Clear Skin through Simple Diet, Exercise, and Lifestyle Changes

Caroline D. Greene

Published by Women's Republic

Atlanta, Georgia USA

WOMEN'S
Republic

ISBN 978-1-48396-790-5

9 781483 967905 >

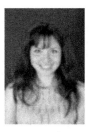

Caroline D. Greene

What Our Readers Are Saying

"MY HORMONES AREN'T THE BOSS ANYMORE!"

★★★★☆Patricia Allen (Throckmorton, TX)

"I JUST WISH I'D FOUND THIS BOOK YEARS AGO"

★★★★★Emily Henderson (Statesboro, GA)

"I'M SO FULL OF ENERGY THAT I'VE ACTUALLY QUIT DRINKING COFFEE"

★★★★★Jenny Brough (Coalgate, OK)

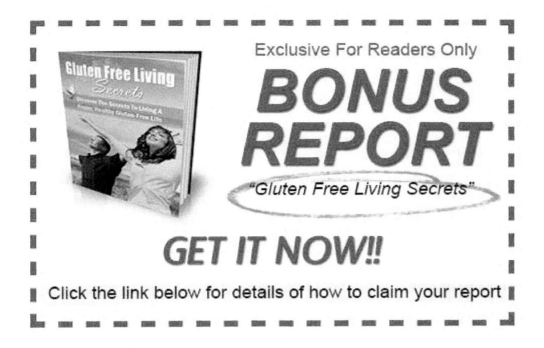
Exclusive Bonus Download: Gluten Free Living Secrets

Are you sick and tired of trying every weight loss program out there and failing to see results? Or are you frustrated with not feeling as energetic as you used to despite what you eat? Perhaps you always seem to have a bit of a " dodgy stomach " and indigestion seems to be a regular part of your life?

There's nothing worse than sitting down to a nice big plate of pasta and enjoying your meal only to be met with a growling stomach and the inevitable rush to the toilet.

It's that bloated feeling you get after eating a piece of bread that just " doesn't seem right " . Almost as if you've eaten something poisonous.

Gluten Free Living Secrets is a complete resource that will tell you everything you need to know about the dangers of eating gluten and how to go about transitioning yourself and your family to a life free of this dangerous substance.

Here's just a taste of what you will discover inside Gluten Free Living Secrets:

- What foods you should focus on when first switching to a gluten-free diet

- The 9 grains that are safe and gluten-free

- The truth about whether you can eat pasta on a gluten-free diet

- What you should know to determine if you have Celiac Disease

- and that's not all...

- Why you may want to consider eliminating gluten from your child's diet

- The top 10 reasons to go gluten-free

- How to transform your pantry to be gluten-free

- A list of essential gluten-free shopping tips

- How to keep your kids happy around their gluten-eating friends

- Tips on staying gluten-free when eating out

Gluten Free Living Secrets comes in a digital PDF format that is easy to read either on your computer or on your eBook reader.

Go to the end of this book for the download link for this Bonus

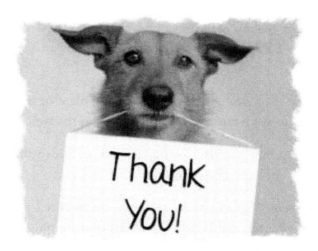

THANK YOU FOR DOWNLOADING MY BOOK. PLEASE REVIEW THIS BOOK ON AMAZON. I NEED YOUR FEEDBACK TO MAKE THE NEXT VERSION BETTER. THANK YOU SO MUCH!

Books by This Author

Permanently Beat Bacterial Vaginosis

Permanently Beat Yeast Infection & Candida

Permanently Beat Urinary Tract Infections

Permanently Beat Hypothyroidism Naturally

Permanently Beat PCOS

The Permanently Beat PCOS Diet & Exercise Shortcuts

The Permanently Beat Hypothyroidism Diet & Exercise Shortcuts

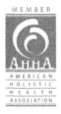

Table of Contents

Disclaimer

While all attempts have been made to provide effective, verifiable information in this Book, neither the Author nor Publisher assumes any responsibility for errors, inaccuracies, or omissions. Any slights of people or organizations are unintentional.

This Book is not a source of medical information, and it should not be regarded as such. This publication is designed to provide accurate and authoritative information in regard to the subject matter covered. It is sold with the understanding that the publisher is not engaged in rendering a medical service. As with any medical advice, the reader is strongly encouraged to seek professional medical advice before taking action.

Chapter 1: Understanding PCOS

What is PCOS?

Maybe you've been exercising and eating healthy, but the numbers on your bathroom scale seem to go up faster than the federal deficit. You've also noticed that your period is acting up, playing hide-and-seek or staying in town for way too long. Why are you gaining so much weight, and what's with your period?

PCOS might be the name for the condition you're facing. PCOS is the short-hand for Polycystic Ovarian Syndrome. It affects nearly 10% of women, some as early as age eleven. Essentially the condition comes from an inability to process insulin normally. Insulin, made by your pancreas, acts as a gatekeeper for glucose to enter your fat, muscle and liver cells. It also inspires your ovaries to produce cells and male and female sex hormones.

Resistance to insulin means high levels of glucose and insulin stay in your system. Your ovaries, like a sink with water left running too long, flood your system with an oversupply of the cells, resulting in excess male and female hormones and sometimes cysts. High levels of insulin also keep fat stores from burning fat as fuel, meaning fat begins to accumulate and your pants get tighter.

Besides weight gain and irregular periods, typical symptoms of PCOS can include cysts (hence the "polycystic" in PCOS), extra facial hair, loss of hair from the scalp, oily skin, acne, and sleep problems. Dark patches and spots on the neck also accompany PCOS. These are caused by higher levels of androgen, which is a sex-related hormone. The condition also brings a risk of infertility, which can be from high insulin levels, delayed ovulation, or other causes. Trickier, hard-to-diagnose symptoms include depression, anxiety, exhaustion, high cholesterol, lower sex drive and lack of alertness.

You might have all of these symptoms, or just a few of them. Even the cysts aren't always a definitive symptom of PCOS.

Even though there is no cure yet for PCOS, you can live a fulfilled, happy life by treating these symptoms and living a lifestyle of regular exercise and healthy diet. One famous example of a successful, healthy woman living with PCOS is Jillian Michaels, the personal trainer and businesswoman with abs that seem carved out of granite. She and thousands of other women do not let PCOS determine their life or their looks.

But before you zoom to your local pharmacy for the latest and greatest pill, consider natural remedies exist that may work just as well. Plus, many of these alternatives may save you considerable cash. Read on for natural tips to get your weight, skin, monthly visit and more back on-track.

7 Warning Signs of PCOS

An ounce of prevention is worth a pound of cure…or in this case, many potential pounds of weight. You can prevent letting your PCOS go untreated by being on the lookout for the warning signs of PCOS. If you read the last section on PCOS and thought, hmm, I've got some of those symptoms, or, no way that's me, check out these signals your body is giving you.

AGE. How old are you? You can dodge this rude question when it comes from precocious children and would-be suitors, but the question needs to be answered honestly here. If you are middle-aged or older, watch your weight. There is a significantly close relationship between being middle-aged or older and overweight to developing PCOS.

TUMMY WEIGHT. Does it seem like your weight settles at your middle and refuses to leave? Women with PCOS carry the majority of their fat in their midsection. Typically weight is displaced throughout multiple parts of the body, such as the upper arms, butt, stomach, thighs and chest, but if fat seems to clearly prefer your stomach, that could be a sign of PCOS.

SKIN TAGS AND DARK SKIN PATCHES. These tiny pieces of skin are harmless, flesh-colored or slightly darker growths that look like a soft extra piece of skin. Skin tags, or scientifically known as acrochordons, are your skin's version of a hangnail. They can appear anywhere, from your arms, neck, eyelids, groin, breasts, and elsewhere. These pieces of skin do not usually fall off on their own, but you can have a dermatologist remove them. The dark skin patches are different from skin tags. These are called acanthosis nigricans. They are areas which develop patches of thick, dark, velvety skin and noticeable creases. They, too, like skin tags, are harmless.

FREQUENT LIGHT-HEADEDNESS OR DROWSINESS AFTER EATING. After a meal, do you feel dizzy, light-headed or foggy? If you experience those feelings or unusual drowsiness within three hours of eating, that could indicate that you are hypoglycemic. That's a term for when your blood sugar is too low. Extreme cases could cause you to be shaky, have a headache, rapidly-beating heart, nausea and vomiting.

HIGH BLOOD PRESSURE, HYPERTENSION, DIABETES. If you have one of these conditions or another blood lipid abnormality, your risk factor for having PCOS is higher. Each of these conditions is related in the sense that they are each caused by abnormality with glucose and insulin absorption and production.

IRREGULAR PERIODS. When a period stops altogether or is unusually infrequent, PCOS could be the cause. If you normally menstruate on a monthly basis but find that your period pattern has changed significantly, consult your doctor. It could be PCOS or another cause.

RELATIVE WITH PCOS. If you have a mother, sister, aunt, grandmother or another close relative who has been diagnosed with PCOS, the odds are higher for you to have this condition as well. Ask your family privately so you can be aware of what you are genetically predisposed to.

Pop Quiz on PCOS

If you've noticed that some of the symptoms in the previous section apply to you and your body, take the quiz below to see if you have PCOS. This is one quiz you don't want to do well on. At least if you score high, you'll know the next step is to see a doctor for an official diagnosis, and then you can take further steps to receive treatment to lessen your symptoms.

Periods

Do you experience unusual, irregular bleeding?

Do you have less than eight periods in a year?

Have you gone longer than four months without a period?

Have you been struggling to get pregnant?

Hair

Have you noticed hair growth on your body that typically a man would have, such as on the chest, stomach, upper arms, back, sideburns, and neck area?

Has the hair on your scalp been thinning?

Skin

Has your acne been a persistent problem, or even increased as you have become an adult despite treatment?

Weight

Has your weight increased significantly?

Does your weight seem to be primarily gathered at your stomach?

Have you felt that regular exercise and eating healthy has not resulted in any weight loss?

Do you feel light-headed or drowsy within three hours after eating?

Family

Do you know of a close relative who has diabetes, PCOS, or another blood lipid-related disorder?

If you answered yes to over five of these questions, you need to visit a doctor for confirmation of whether you have a diagnosis of PCOS. These symptoms may not go away on their own. Ask your relatives if they have a history of PCOS so you can inform your doctor if you have a family history of this condition.

The Causes of PCOS

Sometimes when you get an unwelcome diagnosis, the first thing you want to do is find out why this happened to you. Did you eat something strange? Is it in the family genes? If you took the quiz in the last section and answered "Yes" to over five questions, then you may have gone to a doctor to be tested for PCOS, or Polycystic Ovarian Syndrome.

Even though placing blame is not going to be as helpful to you as seeking treatment, it is important to look at the causes of PCOS. Understanding the reasons and triggers can help you understand your own symptoms, as well as support others who may be facing the same diagnosis.

There may be more than one cause of PCOS, which is why the symptoms vary so much from woman to woman. Scientists and doctors continue to study each case for clues as to why some women are more genetically vulnerable to developing PCOS, and why some seem to develop it after certain lifestyle choices. Even though the inherited-nature of PCOS has been established by scientific studies, no single gene or set of genes has been identified as the culprit for causing or contributing to PCOS.

Here are the most commonly agreed-upon causes:

- Defect in the hypothalamus, which is an almond-sized area in the brain just above the brain stem. This defect leads to intense LH pulses that trigger the ovaries to make more and more male hormones. These LH pulses are usually the green light for your ovaries to ovulate and create the corpus luteum, which is the early stage of the lining of blood within your uterus. That is why the pulses are called LH pulses, short for "Luteinizing Hormone." With your ovaries going full speed ahead making testosterone, it's no wonder that symptoms such as male-patterned hair growth appear.

- Ovaries are producing abnormal testosterone. If your ovaries are making testosterone with abnormal enzymes, it may be affecting the appearance and functionality of your body in ways that it normally wouldn't.

- Insulin resistance that leads to high insulin levels. The high level of insulin can also increase the intensity of the pulses in the hypothalamus, meaning more male hormones are produced.

- Genetic causes. The rate of having PCOS if a close relative has it is much higher than if you aren't related to someone with PCOS. It could be genes or lifestyle, but the correlations are undeniable. Forty percent of women who have PCOS also have a sister who has it, and slightly fewer women with PCOS also share the condition with their mom.

The important facts to take away about the causes of PCOS are what can you do to prevent getting it yourself or helping others to avoid this diagnosis. Managing your weight through diet and exercise is a key part of avoiding this condition, because heavier weight can trigger the syndrome or increase the severity of its symptoms. If you know that PCOS runs in your family, then you can visit your doctor regularly to ensure that your insulin and glucose are functioning at a normal level. The more you take ownership of your health and increase your own awareness, the more likely you'll catch conditions like PCOS early on and be able to prevent or alleviate major symptoms.

Emotional Effects of PCOS

The visible effects of PCOS make it one of the most emotionally frustrating hormone disorders out there. Obesity, in an era where ads, movies and billboards make being skinny the pinnacle of success, is hard. The excessive hair growth in areas where men would typically have hair can cause women with PCOS to feel self-conscious and unfeminine. For women who are seeking to get pregnant, the lack of ovulation and infertility can seem like an unfair, insurmountable challenge. Girls as young as age ten or eleven who get PCOS can be overwhelmed by cruel jokes at school and by siblings for severe facial acne and being overweight.

Dealing with these kinds of symptoms would harm any woman's self-esteem and sense of self-beauty. Feeling like a healthy, beautiful woman is hard enough without these added health issues.

Battling these symptoms can leave you feeling depressed, exhausted, and ashamed. You'll notice this by a depressed mood, difficulty sleeping, loss of interest in favorite activities, exhaustion, and changes in appetite. Women with PCOS seem to be the most distressed by the excessive facial and body hair, scalp hair loss, irregular periods, and difficulty conceiving. Many women say that having no period made them feel childlike and experiencing unwanted hair growth made them feel less feminine. Even the famed health and fitness celebrity Jillian Michaels hesitated to speak about her struggles with PCOS for fear that people would think she was unhealthy!

It's important to realize if you have PCOS, you are not alone. There are many women who gain strength from each other as they face this condition together. If you can find a support group that meets to discuss PCOS, you may be reassured by what you learn and hear. If you can't find a local group, search online for a PCOS support web site. Sites such as pcosupport.org could be a source of encouragement and awareness of symptoms and treatments for you. Message boards, newsletters, testimonials and even books written by women with PCOS can provide insights that only others with PCOS can share. You may be able to connect with some of these women and ask questions or share your experiences. You can learn about new treatments and research.

A quick side-note about contributing information on these sites: Be careful not to share information that could allow someone to identify your full name, address, social security number or other personal information. Even though the majority of people accessing these sites are friendly folk who are seeking answers like you are, there are some who take advantage of emotionally-distressed people on websites. Stay anonymous, and you can still learn and share what you need about PCOS.

Much of the depression and anxiety you may feel if you have PCOS is due to the hormonal imbalance that comes with the condition. Psychological tests have shown that women with PCOS have higher levels of cortisol, which is a stress hormone, compared with women who do not have PCOS. You may notice this can cause frustration, sensitivity, obsessive-compulsive behavior, aggressiveness, reduced feeling of satisfaction with sex life, and a feeling of being unattractive.

If you are beginning to notice these emotions and feelings in yourself or in someone you know with PCOS, seek treatments that are will help you to lessen the effects of these symptoms. Healthy diet and exercise can boost your endorphins and help you to feel healthy and good about yourself. Taking a supplement or pill to lower the levels of male hormones in your system may slow the effects of hair growth and help you to ovulate again.

Chapter 2: Negative Effects of Living with PCOS

Becoming Pregnant Despite Higher Rate of Infertility with PCOS

Many women struggle with infertility as a result of Polycystic Ovarian Syndrome. If you recall the section on the emotional impact of PCOS on women, then you know that depression, anxiety, and other negative psychological changes can be symptoms of the condition. Infertility is one of the leading complaints from women to their doctors about PCOS. The good news is many women with PCOS can still become pregnant without any medical assistance. If you are having difficulty getting pregnant, consider all the other factors that could be responsible and have your partner checked out as well.

PCOS is known to cause infertility, and so if you are interested in having a baby, get ready to take some steps that will prepare your body for its best chances at conceiving. Most treatment plans for PCOS emphasize the importance of regular exercise and treatments for the regulation and production of insulin to bring back regular ovulation for eventual pregnancy. Metformin, a medicine used to help control the amount of glucose in blood and increase sensitivity to insulin, can help. In fact, many IVF programs prescribe metformin in a variety of forms for women, because it can help with successful implantation of the embryo in the uterus.

If you have PCOS and your goal is to get pregnant, consider the following steps to take:

- Drop some pounds if you are overweight. This is the best way to start. Even if it's only 2-5 pounds off of your body, your hormones will be more likely to kick in and start your period again. If you aren't normally active, start small, by taking stairs and walking. Have a goal, like 30 minutes per day. Many women say they are too busy for exercise, and that their job and/or children don't allow them the time to work out. But here's the secret: even if it's only ten minutes, take a walk. Every little bit helps to increase your metabolism and get your blood flowing. You want to prepare your body to be at its best for the strain that pregnancy will put on it.

- Ask your gynecologist about a medication that will lower insulin. If your insulin levels decrease and you are exercising, you'll have a better opportunity to begin ovulating. Ovulation (with sexual activity, of course!) can lead to a higher likelihood of pregnancy.

- Consider hormone therapy, such as birth control. With PCOS, your hormones are out-of-whack. Higher and lower in a constantly changing cycle that disrupts ovulation and causes some of the changes to your appearance. To regulate your roller-coaster of sex hormones, a hormonal birth control may be a good option. There is another excellent reason for taking birth control to get your period back: if the endometrial lining in your uterus stays put for too long, it can increase your risk of uterine cancer. When you have your period, that lining sloughs off, which is why you bleed. But if the lining stays in your body, uterine cancer can develop. Additionally, birth control may be able to help with decreasing acne and the excessive hair growth.

- Monitor your ovulation. Ovulating is key to becoming pregnant, and unfortunately with PCOS, having a period does not always mean you are releasing an egg. You can confirm that you are ovulating by three types of tests: home kits that measure the LH, or luteinizing hormone pulse; thermometers to measure and record basal body temperature on a daily basis; and lab tests for your progesterone blood level. The lab test is likely to be the most reliable compared with basal body temperature or home kits.

- Toss the cigarettes if you are a smoker. Smoking can actually keep the level of androgens, the sex hormones, higher in your body.

Try these steps as you continue your attempts to become pregnant. It may take time and changes to your normal habits, but it may be possible for you to conceive, even with PCOS.

Risk Factors for PCOS: Increased Chance of Diabetes, High Blood Pressure, Miscarriages, Eating Disorders and Uterine Cancer

Having Polycystic Ovarian Syndrome does mean that you are at a higher risk for other hormone- and insulin-related disorders and conditions. From previous chapter, you may remember that PCOS symptoms are mainly attributable to being insulin-resistant. This insulin-resistance affects your body in a myriad of ways that increase your risk of developing diabetes, high blood pressure, having miscarriages, eating disorders, and uterine cancer.

These conditions are not inevitable. In fact, there are many steps you can take to help lower your chances of developing these disorders. First, let's talk about each of them and why they are related to PCOS:

DIABETES

Diabetes and PCOS are strongly correlated, meaning if you have PCOS, your chances of developing diabetes as well are significantly high. Studies have shown that over half of women with PCOS will develop diabetes or pre-diabetes before they turn forty.

HIGH BLOOD PRESSURE, ALSO CALLED HYPERTENSION

Developing high blood pressure can happen with or without PCOS, but your chances of developing it if you have PCOS are greater. High blood pressure brings many risks, including heart attacks. Women with PCOS are four to seven times more likely to have a heart attack than women without PCOS.

If you are pregnant after following the steps in the previous section, it's important to realize that high blood pressure can complicate a pregnancy. One type of high blood pressure called pre-eclampsia has risk factors that put women with PCOS at risk: high blood pressure before pregnancy and type 2 diabetes.

MISCARRIAGES

Tragically, women with PCOS have three times the normal risk of miscarrying, especially during the early months of pregnancy. However, in the section about becoming pregnant despite the risk of infertility with PCOS, studies have shown that women can conceive even with PCOS. To avoid miscarrying, team up with your gynecologist and endocrinologist to protect you and your baby-to-be by monitoring you and your fetus's insulin and glucose levels.

During pregnancy, the placenta provides nourishment to the fetus, such as blood sugar. Insulin is not shared. If the mother has PCOS and a high level of blood sugar, the fetus will receive excessive blood sugar, causing rapid weight gain, just as it does to adult females. To avoid this happening to your baby-to-be, monitor your blood sugar levels carefully before and during the pregnancy. Disciplined dieting will help you protect the fetus from abnormal development or being miscarried.

EATING DISORDERS

The rapid weight gain and predisposition toward putting weight on around the stomach area can cause many women with PCOS to develop eating disorders such as bulimia and anorexia. Those women who developed PCOS earlier in life and may not have realized that their weight gain was due to PCOS seem to be at particular risk. Some have starved themselves or over-exercised in the extreme in an effort to lose the weight. Frustration with the slow progress and feeling unhealthy can lead to low self-esteem and depression, which some women react to by emotional overeating. Unfortunately these types of eating and exercise behaviors can aggravate PCOS symptoms by putting the body's hormones and blood sugar levels out-of-whack. If you know your eating habits are not healthy or recognize those behaviors in someone who has PCOS, consult a nutritionist and/or psychologist. These behaviors can damage your body by depriving it of the nutrients it needs. You can lose the weight by taking the right kinds of insulin- and glucose-regulators, engaging in regular exercise at the right intensity, and other steps. If you feel out of control, contact your primary physician or a nutrition professional as soon as possible. Don't be ashamed to seek help, because your body's health is at stake.

UTERINE OR ENDOMETRIAL CANCER

The high levels of male hormones resulting from PCOS and the likelihood of not ovulating, or anovulation, can mean that you have fewer periods. When you have a period, the progesterone hormone in your body signals that the endometrial lining in your uterus has to go. The lining is in-place to provide nutrients to a growing fetus, and your body knows that if there is no fetus there, the lining should be shed. When you have PCOS, your body continues producing estrogen, but it does not produce progesterone as it should. Without progesterone, you skip your period and that lining stays in your uterus. The longer it stays, the thicker it becomes, which is a condition called endometrial hyperplasia. As a result, you become at risk of developing uterine or endometrial cancer.

To prevent this from happening, keep record of your periods. If you notice that you have not had a period for over four months or that you have less than eight periods during a year, inform your doctor. They may suggest you begin taking a form of birth control or natural progesterone injections that will regulate your hormones. The bottom line is, having your period is actually helpful to your body, because it rids it regularly of the lining.

Chapter 3: Diagnosing PCOS

What PCOS Isn't

Receiving a diagnosis for PCOS means that certain other hormonal disorders have been ruled out. PCOS is a diagnosis of exclusion, meaning that other conditions are considered first, and if it isn't those conditions, then it may be PCOS. In fact, 10-15% of women who appear to have PCOS actually have a different type of hormonal disorder.

So before you convince yourself that your symptoms are clearly indicative of PCOS, consult your doctor, preferably an endocrinologist. Ask about the possibility of these other hormonal disorders causing your symptoms.

HAIRAN syndrome

Appropriately-acronymed, HAIRAN syndrome deals primarily with excess body hair. It also has accompanying symptoms of insulin resistance and skin pigmentation. These symptoms are all similar to those PCOS causes. The difference is in how the insulin resistance originates; if it is HAIRAN syndrome, then changes occur during puberty, and if it is PCOS, it can occur at any time from age 10 through late twenties.

Congenital and adult-onset adrenal hyperplasia

This long-winded hormonal disorder causes similar symptoms to PCOS. Tests will show high levels of the male hormone testosterone in women. This disorder isn't common, but it does tend to run in some Jewish, Eskimo and Hispanic families.

Idiopathic hirsutism.

What's with all the hair? It may be PCOS, but it might also be idiopathic hirsutism. This condition causes excessive hair growth for no apparent reason. Some of these women have raised testosterone levels, but some do not. Menstrual cycles may not be affected at all.

Cushing's syndrome

Rapid weight gain of over 25 pounds in one year can seem like PCOS, but it may be Cushing's syndrome. In this condition, high blood pressure, stretch marks from weight gain, a fat pad on the back of the neck, acne, hirsutism, and lack of periods can all be caused by too much cortisol. Cortisol is a stress hormone produced by the adrenal glands. This condition is often mistaken for PCOS.

Thyroid abnormality

If the thyroid part of your brain is hyper- or hypoactive, then major changes in your metabolism, menstrual cycles, and hair loss may occur. Underactive thyroids can result in heavy menstrual cycles, while overactive thyroids can mean periods stop. The thyroid is directly related to your energy level and heartbeat rapidity, and any abnormality in how it functions is often the result of a hormonal imbalance.

High level of prolactin

Seven to 20% of women with PCOS can also have a high level of prolactin. This hormone triggers milk production and progesterone production after having a baby. Your pituitary gland is the culprit in this condition, and its overabundance of prolactin can cause your period to be off-cycle or absent, hair growth and loss, and acne.

Ovarian hyperthecosis

Ultrasound tests may reveal women's ovaries to be thick. High testosterone and insulin resistance can also be symptoms of this condition. Women can have ovarian hyperthecosis and PCOS simultaneously.

Because PCOS is a diagnosis of exclusion, it is important to weigh these other conditions as possibilities as well. Your doctor can run tests to determine the cause of your symptoms. You've already taken a positive step forward by observing your symptoms. The earlier you detect your symptoms and seek treatment, the better chance you have of alleviating symptoms and avoiding more serious conditions such as diabetes or a heart attack.

Typical Tests for PCOS

If you're curious to know how your doctor knows you have PCOS, here's some insider knowledge. Typical tests for PCOS include a standard medical history, in which your doctor quizzes you on your period pattern, any recent weight changes, and other symptoms. He or she should also ask you if you have any relatives who have PCOS or another insulin- or hormone-related disorder.

Your doctor will conduct a physical exam, measuring your blood pressure and checking for physical signs of PCOS. These signs can include excessive male-patterned hair growth, proportionally more weight at your middle, and swollen ovaries, which can indicate the presence of cysts. Before your appointment, you may want to consider taking a break from shaving or waxing to let your hair grow naturally. This will allow the doctor to get a better understanding of whether the hair growth is related to PCOS or another cause. Hopefully you can schedule your appointment around a time when you won't have to wear a swimsuit!

During an appointment, your doctor or the nurse may draw some of your blood to test it. They will send samples through a battery of tests to check the levels of androgen, glucose and insulin. These tests may take a few days to return, but they are more reliable than a simple physical exam.

If your periods seem to have taken a long vacation but other symptoms of PCOS are not evident, your doctor may take a vaginal ultrasound, also known as a sonogram. Essentially this test is when sound waves are used to photograph your pelvic area, ovaries and uterus. The resulting photograph may show cysts and swelling of the ovaries.

PCOS symptoms are different for every woman with the condition. The degree of weight gain, scalp hair loss, hair growth on the body and other physical changes can vary. Each of these symptoms can also be related to a condition that isn't PCOS. Because of the variation and potential other causes, your doctor may need to conduct multiple tests. Don't be afraid to get a second opinion if you aren't sure about the diagnosis.

When you know your diagnosis, you have already taken the first step in recovering control over your health. In the upcoming chapter on the steps to easing your symptoms through diet, exercise, supplements and more, you'll learn about what you can do to prevent further symptoms and regulate your hormones and insulin.

Chapter 4: Treating PCOS

Supplements

The praises for the benefits of supplements often go unsung by doctors and nurses, but many of these herbal, natural supplements can help you regulate and ease your symptoms. Herbal supplements can be hit-or-miss, as they affect different bodies in different ways. However, many women who have PCOS have tried the following supplements with great success.

Herbal supplements which contain vital nutrients that affect you body in similar ways as pharmaceutical pills are sometimes nicknamed "nutraceuticals." These supplements can help your body produce and respond to insulin. Sometimes foods do not have a high concentration of the necessary nutrients to treat PCOS, and so supplements provide that higher concentration.

Katie Humphrey, one woman who uses nutraceuticals to treat her PCOS, has written about her trials and successes with herbal supplements in her book, "Nutraceuticals: My Secret Weapon". She writes, "Natural supplements are closest to their original state as a whole food so they are recognized and properly utilized by the body." She says that selecting the best types of herbal supplements for her body has allowed her to regulate her periods and improve her digestion. By choosing a more naturally-made supplement rather than a pill, you are strengthening your body to deal with many of the symptoms on its own and forgoing some detrimental side-effects in the process.

Here are some of the top recommended-supplements for treating symptoms of PCOS:

Helps control insulin or glucose levels:

Biotin, carnitine, chromium, cinnamon, D-chiro-inositol, D-Pinitol, fish oil, green tea, gymnema, inositol, magnesium, multi-vitamin/mineral, NAC, Vitamin D, zinc

Helps with weight-loss by suppressing the appetite:

5-hydroxy-tryptophan, carnitine, CLA (Conjugated Linoleic Acid, from meat and dairy products), d-Pinitol, fish oil, green tea, inositol, magnesium, multi-vitamin/mineral, Vitamin D

Helps with hair loss:

Biotin, carnitine, fish oil, green tea, Vitex (chasteberry), zinc, saw palmetto, multi-vitamin/mineral

Helps with acne:

Fish oil, green tea, inositol, multi-vitamin/mineral, saw palmetto, Vitex (chasteberry)

Improves fertility and helps to regulate hormones:

D-chiro-inositol, d-Pinitol, fish oil, green tea, Indole 3 carbanol, Inositol, saw palmetto, natural progesterone, multi-vitamin/mineral, Vitamin D, Vitex (chasteberry)

Some supplements rumored to alleviate symptoms of PCOS are licorice, Vanadyl sulfate, Momordica, Quercetin, Vitamin B6, and Slentiva, but it is not yet proven whether these have consistently positive effects on women with PCOS.

If you noticed that some of the supplements are in multiple categories, that is because some supplements carry multiple benefits. Green tea, fish oil and Vitamin D are three of the most common supplements that help women with PCOS in a variety of ways, and each of these can be found at your local pharmacy or grocery store. You may prefer trying these more affordable, commonplace supplements before paying the big bucks for specialty herbal supplements. As you try them, you'll find what works for your body. Always research what the recommended amount to ingest is and potential allergies before consuming them, just to be on the safe side.

Supplements are called supplements for a reason. They back up your main form of treatment, whether it is healthy diet and exercise, birth control pills, or other forms of insulin and glucose regulators. Try these supplements and see what works for you. You may end up saving quite a bit of cash in the end and avoiding having to take pills with major side effects.

C'mon, Cinnamon!

Spice up your life and your meals with a little cinnamon. This spice has many benefits for women dealing with PCOS. Here are some of the pros to partaking in a bit of cinnamon:

- Helps your body burn carbs faster

- Reduces blood glucose levels

- Increases insulin sensitivity

- Decreases testosterone levels

- Regularizes your period

The reason it works is that cinnamon as an insulin sensitizer. In 2003, the National Institutes of Health conducted a study that showed improvement for people who have type 2 diabetes when they included cinnamon in their diet.

Cinnamon also has many other health benefits. It is thought to improve your memory, aid digestion, suppress bacteria and lower your cholesterol. The dietary mixture cinnamaldehyde has been shown to activate antioxiodants and even work against melanoma, leukemia and lymphoma. Because of its ability to help your brain function, studies are ongoing to see whether cinnamon helps Alzheimer's patients.

So how do you introduce cinnamon into your diet as more than just a sprinkled topping? Lucky for you, it's got as many forms as Spanx. You can take cinnamon as a pill of about 200 to 300 milligrams. You can sip cinnamon tea. You can use 1-2 teaspoons of its powdered form in your daily cooking. Toss some on your cereal or toast at breakfast.

Cinnamon comes from the bark of the Cinnamon tree in Southeast Asia. For centuries it has been regarded as a spice with special properties. In the Proverbs, a book of the Bible, a lover's bed is perfumed with cinnamon, and cinnamon was used in incense for the temple. The ancient Egyptians and Greeks used cinnamon in their offerings to the gods, saving it for special occasions because of how expensive and rare it was.

Today, you can buy all the cinnamon you want at your local grocery store or market. But how much should you take for its effects to be significant, and how much is too much? People who have taken more than a half teaspoon at one time have said they suffered bowel irritation, increased heart rate, uterine contractions (because cinnamon can actually be used to induce contractions in pregnant women), blood thinning, and kidney and liver problems. However, that is only in the case when you are taking high doses of cinnamon. Small, gradually-consumed amounts can help you lower your blood sugar significantly.

Most doctors will tell you that you can take about 200-300 mg of cinnamon extract, or 1-6 g of powdered cinnamon each day for forty days.

Important note: Some companies sell a spice called "cassia" under the name cinnamon, even though it is not true cinnamon. Cassia contains higher amounts of coumarin, which is a compound that can negatively affect your kidney and liver. Check the label of your source of cinnamon.

Hair Today, Gone Tomorrow

Curly or straight, having hair where you want it is great. Seventy-five percent of women with PCOS notice major changes in their hair growth. PCOS can cause hair from the scalp to fall out. When scalp hair loss is related to the changing levels of androgen hormones due to PCOS, it is called androgenic alopecia. The hair loss is often begins in a triangular shape.

Meanwhile, higher androgen levels can cause male-patterned hair to grow on the abdomen, upper lip, neck, chest, back, thighs, and upper arms. Growing male-like hairs in women is a condition called hirsutism. The coarseness, thickness and color of the hair varies by woman, depending on race and age.

Before you start competing with your boyfriend for the razor to tame your side-burns, consider the fact that many other women and men deal with unwanted hair growth, even if they don't have PCOS. As a result, pharmacies are always stocked with affordable, do-it-yourself hair removal products.

Here are some natural remedies for this hairy situation to help you avoid feeling like a bald Elvis:

Temporary hair removal

- Waxing or sugaring, which pulls hair out by its follicles or roots

- Lotions such as Nair

- Threading

- Bleaching

- Shaving

- Depilatories, which remove hair chemically

- Tweezers or rotary epilators, which are hair removal devices

- Topical prescription creams

Permanent hair removal

- Electrolysis, in which an electric current zaps the hair root, removing hair permanently

- Laser hair removal, in which a laser beam destroys the hair follicle

Even though some manufacturers may claim that their cream removes hair permanently, don't believe it. Topical creams do not remove hair permanently, although other methods (electrolysis, laser hair removal) can.

Now, for the top of your head. Most women lose a fourth of their hair before they start feeling the wind on their scalp. If you have been diagnosed with PCOS, you may want to go ahead and try some of the techniques below for keeping your hair thick. To keep your locks long and lustrous, here are key tips.

- Consume vitamins that will help your hair. Your hair follicles need minerals such as Vitamin B-6, folate, Vitamin C, Vitamin E, zinc, sulfur, magnesium and biotin.

- Mix two tablespoons of oat float into your conditioner. This flour has lipids that can thicken individual strands of your hair, giving you a fuller look.

- Rub aromatherapy oils into your scalp. Oils made from lavender, jojoba, grapeseed, thyme, rosemary and cedarwood may help stimulate hair growth.

- For the truly adventurous, massage a raw egg into your hair. Rinse it thoroughly after 5-10 minutes. Eggs are rich in proteins that can make your hair stronger.

- Don't distress your tresses. Avoid pulling your hair into a tight ponytail. Set your hairdryer, curler or flat iron to the lowest settings, or skip using them. Select natural hair products that don't use harsh chemicals.

For more information on specific remedies for hair removal and hair thickening, visit www.hairfacts.com for honest advice on a wide range of hair-related products.

Healthy Diet

Eating a healthy diet and exercising are possibly the very best actions you can take to reduce your PCOS symptoms. A PCOS-healthy diet is slightly different than your garden-variety healthy woman's diet.

CHOOSE YOUR MENU WISELY

The best diet for you if you're dealing with PCOS is lean proteins, whole grain, fruits and veggies. Keep your dairy intake low. Green vegetables such as cabbage, celery, spinach, broccoli, green beans, artichokes and asparagus provide your body with antioxidants that boost your body's immunity.

You want to avoid processed food and sugars. Lessening the amount of blood sugar means you're helping to keep those glucose levels down, which are causing your ovaries to work overtime and your fat cells to keep the fat inside instead of burning it.

MAKE FREQUENT BUT SMALLER MEALS

Keep your blood sugar down to a normal level by planning 4-6 smaller meals each day.

Eating more frequently will keep your metabolism higher, assisting you in burning fat at a higher rate. Your portion size is critical, though – if you are eating larger meals more often, your body may be taking in more glucose than it can handle well.

Try not to skip out on your meals, or your planned snacks. When you skip these, you'll tend to binge when it is the next time to eat. You'll be hungrier, so your inhibitions will be lowered. You'll be more likely to go for the chocolate chip cookies you would have skipped if you'd had your lunch as usual.

LOSE THE BOOZE

Every time you raise your glass in a cheer with the girls, you're consuming hundreds of empty calories. When you drink alcohol, you know your inhibitions are lowered. That means you're more likely to be tempted to obey your cravings for meat lover's pizza. Also, if you are taking insulin or glucose regulating medicine, alcohol may affect the performance of those medicines, rendering them less effective.

H20: HERE WE GO

While your martini glasses are taking a break, fill up your water bottle with good, clear H20. When you drink water before a meal, you can burn more calories. Drinking water will also prevent dehydration, which can cause your skin to look pale. When you're dehydrated, you feel weak, and that means you'll be less likely to exercise or do your other important tasks.

MAKE VITAMINS PART OF YOUR PLAN

Multivitamins are vital for a balanced diet. In the previous chapter on supplements, you learned about the incredible benefits of multi-vitamins. Compare the labels of various bottles on the shelf to choose one designed to give you the nutrients you need. For example, B-12, folic acid, calcium, and iron are especially important for good skin, hair, and nail health.

PUT BUTTER ON THE BENCH

Cook smart by substituting the dairy-heavy ingredients to your meals with low-fat alternatives. Use a cooking spray like Pam instead of butter or oil. Use lowfat milk or soy milk instead of 2% or whole milk.

You'll find that by following these simple rules, you can increase your weight loss and the overall health of your body.

Oily Skin and Acne

You've been diagnosed with PCOS, and now it feels like your skin is breaking out into more zits, whiteheads and pimples than a pubescent 13-year-old. What can you do to clear up your skin, and why is your skin suddenly so oily?

The increased level of hormones in your skin is directly related to your skin's excess oils. It's usually the male hormones that are responsible for severe acne that resists dermatological treatment. Essentially the hair follicles skin secret an oil called sebum that comes up through your skin's pores. When the pore's opening is stopped up by oil and bacteria, pimples and blackheads form. When many follicles become stopped up, this creates the appearance of multiple pimples, or acne.

Mild acne is normal for women from adolescence. When it continues to be an issue through a woman's mid-twenties, then it is more likely to be caused by PCOS. Severe acne is when the pimples become inflamed. Fewer than 1 in 100 Caucasian women under 21 have severe acne, so it is not nearly as common as mild acne. The good news is that mild to moderate acne is not usually hard to reverse. Let's talk about what you can do to help your skin heal and prevent pizza-face.

WHAT TO DO:

Eat healthy foods that contain less sugar and grease. These foods are not only essential for your health, but they will help you avoid excess oils developing on your skin.

Consider oral contraceptives as a way to regulate your hormones. These can reduce male hormones, which are responsible for increasing the oil your skin is secreting. If you are already on an oral contraceptive, talk with your doctor about switching to another kind, and let them know you are interested in a type that will help you against your acne.

Androgens are a major factor in your PCOS symptoms, so you may want to consider using an antiandrogen, such as spironolactone. Aldactone is one brand-name for this drug. Women who take this drug tend to see an improvement over the next 60 to 90 days. Always ask your doctor about the side effects of a drug such as Aldactone, as it can affect your plans to be pregnant, give you headaches, breast tenderness, increased urinary frequency and potentially a reduced sex drive.

For severe acne, your doctor may give you a prescription for Accutane or Benzaclin. Both of these can dry out your lips, hair and skin. These drugs can be very effective in clearing up your skin, but they may take up to four or six months to begin working noticeably.

WHAT TO AVOID:

Skip the squeeze. When you pinch or squeeze the pimples, you are damaging your skin, opening it up to infection, and increasing your risk of scarring. It doesn't help, no matter how tempting it might be!

Select acne-friendly sunscreens and lotions. Some lotions and sunscreens are made with many types of oils that can irritate your skin and increase acne. Check the label before you buy a bottle and see if it is a non-comedogenic product, which means it's unlikely to worsen your acne.

Watch the washing. Too much hard-scrubbing and overly-frequent washing can aggravate your acne. It can remove necessary oils that your skin needs along with the excess oil, and that can leave your skin dry and cracking. Limit washing your face to three times per day. When you use soap and water, hot compresses, astringents, and try to avoid using your fingers (which carry oils and dirt) on your acne, then you can keep the acne from becoming inflamed. But the only way to stop new acne from developing is by using some of the measures described above.

Battling Weight Gain

Remember studying wars in history class? The generals who won their wars didn't win by saying oh, it'll all work out. They didn't send their solders into battle without armor and weapons. No, they had a plan.

When you have PCOS and your body processes food differently than other women's bodies, you are going to need a plan. You'll need the right resources to win, such as exercise equipment, fitting athletic gear, a heart monitor, good shoes, and more. You are now a general of your own health and fitness against the weight-gaining forces of PCOS.

We're not saying you're going to have to pack up some ammo and hunt the jungle to fight someone to lose weight (although hiking is definitely a great form of exercise!). Your battle is against your weight gain, and the victor will be determined by your level of discipline in diet and exercise.

Remember, an army marches on its stomach. So as we go through key exercise tips that will help you win your battle against weight gain, keep following the healthy eating tactics I covered in the previous section. Eating nutritious foods in the proper portion size will you energized and empowered to stick to your exercise plan!

Now, how to become active if you haven't exercised in a while:

START SMALL IF YOU AREN'T CURRENTLY PHYSICALLY ACTIVE. If you haven't been jogging in a while, you aren't going to want to start out running a marathon. A little bit of exercise can make an incredibly positive difference to your body. Studies have shown that older people who exercised just once a way are 40% less likely to die than people of their same age who do not exercise but only sit.

Some ideas for you: take the stairs instead of the elevator. Walk your dog, or walk with a neighbor who walks their dog. Do jumping jacks or lunges during the commercial breaks of your favorite show.

IF YOU ARE PHYSICALLY ACTIVE, MAKE SURE YOU DOING CARDIO IN YOUR TARGET FAT-BURNING ZONE. What's your target fat-burning zone? We're glad you asked. Your target zone is based on your Target Heart Rate, or THR, which you can find using this formula:

226 – your age x .6 = Target Heart Rate

For example, if you are 35, your target heart rate is 226 – 35 x .6, which equals 114.6. This means your heart rate should be at about 114 or 115 when you are exercising, and that means you are gaining maximum fat burn. Many modern treadmills will tell you your heart-rate if you grip the bars, but a heart-rate monitor is likely to be even more accurate.

MAKE A PLAN. Cardio and strength training six times a week for 45 minutes at a time may sound like what Arnold Schwarzenegger did to get buff, but that is generally accepted as the best way to achieve permanent weight loss. Not everyone can start out at that level of intensity and frequency – in fact, most women need to start at a lower level. Do what's right for you, and write out a plan to gradually build up your level. Keep yourself interested and motivated by mixing up types of exercise. You can do Zumba one day, jogging the next day, and swimming after that. Finding an exercise buddy or selecting a regular class to attend will go a long way. Not only will your exercise be more fun with friends, but they'll also hold you accountable.

Effective Fat-Burning: Your Target Heart Rate

Now that you have an exercise program as outlined in the previous section, "Battling Weight Gain," let's talk about making your workouts really effective. Why walk for hours if you can run for a shorter time and burn the same level of calories?

When you exercise, your heart is pumping oxygenated blood to your muscles to keep them going like the Energizer Bunny. From the lowest heart-rate zone to the highest zone, you are giving your body invaluable benefits, such as a lowered blood pressure, reduced cholesterol, and of course, fat-burn. The sweat is worth it!

Let's look at the zones so you can see where you need to be. The best way to check and see if you are in your preferred zone as you exercise is by using a heart monitor.

Healthy Heart Zone – 50-60% of your maximum heart rate. This zone is great if you are just returning to being active. You'll achieve all the benefits we just discussed and even lower your chance of degenerative diseases in the future, such as Alzheimer's. That's right – as your body stays fit, your mind is more likely to stay sharp! Plus, get ready for this: you burn 85% fat at this level. Eight-five percent is obviously a very high percentage, but the total amount of calories you burn may not be as high as another zone. So if you want to max your percentage and the total amounts, take a look at these other zones.

Fat-Burning Zone – 60-70% of your maximum heart rate. The raised intensity level continues to burn your fat at 85% but burns more total calories. That's a win-win!

Aerobic Zone – 70-80% of your maximum heart rate. You are working on your endurance at this zone. Your heart will become stronger, allowing you to perform at a higher level. You'll burn 50% from fat.

Anaerobic Zone – 80-90% of your maximum heart rate. Wow, you are an athlete! At this rate, you are burning up oxygen at the highest level you can during exercise. In future workouts, you'll resist fatigue better and be able to work out for a longer period of time. You don't burn as many calories from fat, however – just 15%.

Maximum Heart Rate – 90-100% of your heart rate. Competing in the Olympics? Sprinting for a gold medal? You are working as hard as your heart will allow and burning the highest number of calories. Be careful of going at this intensity. Many who are not trained athletes can injure their bodies and overwork their heart. Save this for the races when it counts.

Each of these rates has a right time and place, depending on your exercise routine. Switch it up for a stronger heart and more effective workout. Remember to pace yourself and build up gradually so you can work out longer and burn more calories from fat.

Now that you know the various levels of heart rate intensity and how that helps you burn fat, how can you raise your metabolic rate? See the next section on raising your metabolic rate to find out.

Raise Your Metabolic Rate

Raise your rate! Your metabolic rate, that is. When you increase the rate at which you burn calories, your workouts will be more effective. You'll be further along on your way to the weight loss you want.

It's a fact that as you grow older, your metabolism slows down. When you don't burn off the calories you've consumed, they are converted into fat for later use. But there are many small, daily actions you can take to raise your metabolism and then let your body burn calories even when you're resting.

Key pointers for boosting that magic ratio:

EAT FREQUENT SMALL MEALS. Yes, eat more often! You probably didn't think you'd hear that in your plan to lose weight. You can eat more often, but the key is smaller portion size. Instead of a sandwich and fruit cup at lunch, try having the sandwich at lunch time and the fruit two to three hours later. What this means is your stomach will be constantly engaging in digestive processes that yes, use energy which means using calories. Make your stomach work! Just be sure that the foods you are consuming are not high in caloric content – choose wisely from among fruits, veggies, lean means and lowfat dairy products.

PACK A HEALTHY SNACK. Snacks like fruit, raisins, nuts and oats can ease your hunger pangs, boost your energy and even raise your metabolism. Go crazy with the Craisins!

DRINK ICED WATER. You make your body work that much harder when you drink cool to cold water. It actually has to expend energy to heat up the water, which means more calories are used up.

EXERCISE AT THE RIGHT HEART RATE. If you read the previous section on your target heart rate, you know that exercising at 60-70% of your maximum heart rate can burn up to 85% of calories from fat. Sustain your exercise at that level for 30 to 45 minutes per day, and you'll be burning calories and boosting your metabolism.

LIFT WEIGHTS. You may have heard that muscle burns more calories than fat does. Long after you lift weights, your muscle cells are still burning calories. They burn calories even when you're asleep!

Dealing with Depression

As your hormones wreak havoc on your body, it is natural to feel a sense of depression. Anxiety is a common symptom of PCOS. After all, you are going through some major changes. Many women feel unattractive as they experience weight gain, unwanted hair growth, scalp hair loss, and acne. They may become sensitive, depressed and aggravated over these symptoms. Typically the best courses of action to improve your mood are weight loss and lower male hormones levels.

But what do you do when no one seems to understand what you are going through?

Here are some steps to preventing depression from getting the best of you.

RECOGNIZE THE SYMPTOMS IN YOURSELF. You'll know that you are depressed if you exhibit some of the following behaviors:

- Sleeping for unusually long hours, or having difficulty sleeping

- Losing interest in hobbies you once enjoyed

- Loss of concentration

- Lowered sex drive

- Negative thoughts about hopelessness, guilt, or even suicide

- Change in appetite: eating either too little or too much

- Distancing yourself from friends and family

When these behaviors have become part of your life, ask for help. Nearly 10% of all Americans experience depression at each year, and many never let others know. When you carry this burden by yourself, you make it harder on yourself than it has to be. You can receive treatment that will allow you to feel like your old self again.

REMEMBER, YOU ARE NOT ALONE. You have family and friends who care about you. All relationships of course are not healthy and fulfilling, and you know which ones those are. Spend time with the people who encourage you and believe in you, and you'll feel more relaxed and able to deal with the stress caused by these changes.

FIND OTHERS WHO ARE AFFECTED BY PCOS. National and local chapters of PCOS-support organizations are filled with other women who are learning to cope with the symptoms of PCOS. Search for PCOSA in your area. Message boards from women like you may have helpful information on new treatments, dealing with infertility, foods which are especially good for you, and other relevant topics. You may befriend some of the other women who have PCOS and be able to encourage them, too. Often these groups offer self-help book recommendations and counseling sessions.

SEEK PSYCHIATRIC TREATMENT. These days, psychiatrists have much better methods of supporting you than asking you to lie on a couch. Psychiatrists can provide you with rapid, effective treatment such as antidepressants. They want you to feel better, and they have considerable training and tools at their disposal to get you feeling like yourself again.

PCOS can affect your mood because of its hormonal changes to your body. The more you learn about its symptoms, the more you will be in control of the level of influence it has on your life. Many women lead successful, fulfilled lives despite the presence of PCOS. You can be one of them as you connect with others who have PCOS and arm yourself with understanding.

Downer Moods Lead to Too Much Food

If you recall the previous section on Dealing with Depression, you already know that anxiety and negative moods can result from the hormonal imbalance and symptoms of PCOS. These feelings of being out of control can manifest themselves in harmful appetite behaviors, such as eating too little or overeating.

Let's talk about overeating. When you feel miserably out of control, like your body is resisting all of your exercise efforts and you aren't sure why your face is breaking out, it's tempting to grab a carton of ice cream and eat your sorrows away.

Unfortunately, this kind of behavior may be satisfying in the short-term, but it will only add to your troubles. As you overeat, you give your body more to process. In women without PCOS, this would simply mean heavier weight gain. But for women with PCOS, this can increase your other symptoms, such as no ovulation, elevated insulin and blood sugar levels, infertility, higher levels of male hormones, hair growth, and scalp hair loss.

You may blame PCOS, and say that your overeating is the fault of the condition. This simply isn't true, because your genes impel you, they don't compel you. You still have control over what you eat, how much you eat, and when you eat it. Take charge of your own health and diet, because no one else will do it for you.

When you are upset and considering eating as much as you possibly can, ask yourself the following questions:

- Why am I feeling so emotional?

- Will eating this really solve the problem that is upsetting me?

- What should the right portion be?

- Is there a healthier version of this snack?

- How much exercise will I need to do later to burn off this food?

Try getting your mind off of food, by removing it from your surroundings. Common sense says that if you have a box of chocolates, popcorn, candy and ice cream within arms' reach, you'll be much more tempted to eat it. So stash it in a place that is difficult to get to. Fill your hunger with a healthy snack that has high volume to calories, such as baby carrots, strawberries, tangerines, or other natural options.

Remember your goals. Write your weight and exercise goals on paper or type them. Then post them in places where you will be likely to look, such as on your fridge door, in your car, in your wallet, or other areas where you will look before you start munching.

If you would like more information on developing healthy eating habits, take some time to read The Thin Commandments, by Dr. Stephen Gullo. This book discusses the glycemic index, abusing food, recipes, dieting and more based on years of counseling women who struggle with eating disorders and weight.

Remember, more is not always better. Go for healthy foods in the right portion sizes. Think smaller meals throughout the day, rather than binge eating.

Chapter 5: Healthy Diet

The Glycemic Index

If you've been diagnosed with PCOS, and you haven't heard of the glycemic index, it's time to introduce you properly.

The glycemic index is a powerful tool for helping you lose weight, maintain a healthy weight, and prevent weight gain. Created in the 1980s, the glycemic index was originally designed to help diabetic people manage their blood sugar. At its core, the glycemic index is simply a scientific method of measuring the impact that specific foods will have on your blood sugar levels. You probably already knew that a chocolate doughnut will raise your blood sugar more than celery, for example.

Like the judges on American Idol, the glycemic index ranks foods. Foods can be labeled on a scale of 0 to 100 on how rapidly they raise your blood sugar. If your blood sugar is going to rocket sky-high, the food will have a higher score. If the type of food will take time to affect your glucose, its score will be lower on the scale.

In general, if a food has a score of 55 or less, that's low. If it's between 56 and 69, that's pretty average. And if its glycemic index is 70 or more, you probably should avoid it.

When you are calculating the total glycemic index of your meal, that's called a glycemic load. Not the most clever name, but it works. You generally want to keep your daily glycemic load under 100.

Here's the magic formula for finding the glycemic load:

glycemic index of food x number of grams of carbs ÷ 100 = glycemic load

For example, if a slice of white bread has a glycemic index of 70, take 70 and multiply it by how many grams of carbohydrates it has. The grams of carbohydrates can be found on the package, so say it is 15 grams. 70 times 15 equals 1,050, then divided by 100 for a glycemic load score of 10.5.

The glycemic index has become an important nutritional tool for women with PCOS. If you would like to try managing your blood sugar with the help of the glycemic index, consider searching for the glycemic index of your food on a mobile app, web site, or purchasing a book on the glycemic index. You can find web sites such as GlycemicGourmet.com, GlycemicIndex.com, or a mobile app such as Glycemic Index Meal Planner.

It may seem like a pain to calculate your food, but it's far more effective for you than carb-counting. For example, one cup of dark cherries and one cup of corn each contain around 15 carbohydrates, give or take. But the blood sugar levels for each are vastly different: those cherries are ranked with a 63 glycemic index, and the corn is only a 48. Because PCOS means your body will be greatly affected by higher levels of blood sugar, you need to aim for those foods with a lower glycemic index. You won't know the better foods for you by looking at the carb count on the nutrition label.

You'll find that using the glycemic index helps you manage your blood sugar, which prevents weight gain. If you keep your blood sugar from raising, your body will produce less insulin, and your muscles can use the insulin more effectively.

Low Glycemic Diet for PCOS

If you recall the previous section, you know about the weight loss and healthy weight maintenance that can come from following the glycemic index. If you are woman with PCOS, you need to focus on regulating your blood sugar, since your body is less sensitive to insulin, which would normally cause that blood sugar to be used up as energy. Lots of blood sugar means lots of weight gain.

So, using the glycemic index to select healthy, satisfying foods that will fill you up and keep blood sugar down is key to preventing bulge. Here are some of the guidelines to a low glycemic diet:

- Select foods from the glycemic index that have high levels of nutrients.

- Limit your carbohydrates. Aim to have 40-50% of your calories from carbs. Most people's diets give them 60% of their calories from carbohydrates, but as a woman with PCOS, you're better off with fewer carbohydrates.

- Eat smaller meals throughout the day, rather than three large ones. This will help you avoid blood sugar spikes after you eat and valleys in-between meals.

- Snack on proteins, like nuts, or another healthy fat source, like avocado.

It's important to understand that using the glycemic index does not mean that you should never eat foods with higher glycemic index scores. You can eat them on occasion if the portion size is minimal. You might be surprised by some foods that have higher effects on your blood sugar, such as potatoes. There are many positive benefits to a food like potatoes, such as potassium, vitamin C, vitamin B6, and more. Just be sure to couple this food with proteins and other low glycemic indexed foods.

Be sure to check the glycemic index of foods before automatically assuming they have a high score. Some will surprise you. Coca-Cola, for example, has a score of 53, because its high fructose corn syrup actually has a low glycemic index, too. Pound cake, bananas, macaroni, instant chocolate pudding, and others are great treats for you, because they won't wreck your blood sugar levels. Just be sure you are keeping them within a reasonable portion size, because the calories and carbohydrates are still considerable, the more you serve.

It's normal that foods contain carbohydrates, and you need them in the right quantities. Your body uses carbohydrates to convert into energy. By using the glycemic index, you can select those foods which will give you the energy you need without the severely high level of glucose. As a woman with PCOS, planning out your meals in advance will probably help you to stick to your weight loss plans and skip the sugary snags.

Lean Meats and Low-Fat Dairy Treats

Moooove over, dairy and fatty meats. We women with PCOS are taking charge of our health and avoiding the pitfalls of foods that create weight gain.

For women with PCOS, our optimal diet is low in saturated fats, low in carbohydrates, moderate in proteins, and as low a glycemic index as possible. Our plates should often look as though they were fresh out of a garden: fresh vegetables, colorful fruits, legumes, and whole grains.

But we all crave savory burgers, chicken wraps and tasty fish from time to time! Red meats give you protein, iron, and calcium. So what's a girl with PCOS to do to avoid those carbs?

Interestingly enough, meat doesn't contain carbohydrates! That's right: chicken, fish, pork, beef, steak – no carbs at all. That means that they are considered outside of the glycemic index. Keep the portion sizes small though, and avoid breading them or adding cracker crumbs. The style of preparation is where the additional carbs come in, with breading, frying, cooking in oil or butter, and other fattening methods that add carbs to the meat.

Fish are fantastic sources of health benefits for your body that you might not get otherwise. The oilier the fish, the more omega-3 fatty acids it contains, which helps your body to reduce inflammation and blood clotting and lower your risk of heart disease. Get this: eating fish just one time per week can lower your risk of a fatal heart attack by forty percent! Again, you want to select oily fish, such as swordfish, salmon, tuna, perch, mackerel, and sardines. But remember not to select those that are prepared with fattening vegetable oil, because that's where the extra carbs sneak their way in. Instead, go for those that are marinated, grilled, or fried with canola oil.

Dairy can be quite contrary. Bur if you select low-fat options, you're saving your body a lot of trouble. Look for fat-free milk and yogurt, because these provide you with calcium and Vitamin D. Their low glycemic index score doesn't hurt, either.

In fact, dairy products, like red meat, provide that much-needed source of calcium for women's bodies. They contain protein, Vitamin B12, zinc, and much more. With a low-fat version or soy milk substitute, you may want to select a product where these vitamins have been added. For example, there are omega-3 enriched eggs that contain much higher levels of those omega-3s than regular eggs.

Get out there and marinate and grill some lean meat! Don't be afraid to include dairy products in your diet, so long as they are low in fat and high in vitamins! You'll feel better and still have those flavors you love.

Getting Fresh with Fish: Salmon, Sardines and Other Seafood

Fish are a tasty, healthful meat that will do your body good. You don't have to scale back on your favorite finned foods when you are planning a PCOS-friendly diet.

You may be saying to yourself, sounds too good to be true. What's the catch of the day?

Lucky for you, landlubber, fish provide valuable vitamins and nutrients for your body. You can lower your risk of a fatal heart attack by 40% if you eat fish just once per week!

When you are staring at the menu or wandering around in the fish market, wondering which to select, consider this: the more oily a fish, the more omega-3 fatty acids it has. Fish such as salmon, sardines, perch, mackerel, tuna and swordfish are recommended as having the highest level of omega-3 fatty acids. These omega-3s, as I covered in a previous section, help your body to reduce blood clotting and inflammation.

Now, a word of caution before you're hooked. Certain types of fish can contain higher levels of mercury. If you are an expectant mommy, then too much mercury can harm the development of your child. This doesn't mean you have to give up your fishy favorites, but you should avoid certain kinds of fish. Swordfish, shark, King mackerel, and tilefish should be on your do-not-eat list, because they tend to live for a longer lifespan and accumulate more mercury than other fish. You can protect yourself by selecting fish that have been raised on a farm, because they are less likely to have mercury.

Now what about crab, lobster, and shrimp, you may ask? Shellfish can be a valuable source of protein for you without carbs or fat.

As I mentioned in the previous section on Lean Meats and Low-Fat Dairy Treats, prepare your food in a way that won't add unnecessary carbohydrates. Frying fish in canola oil will add unwanted carbs, as well cooking it in butter or breading it. Instead, try grilling, marinating, or baking your seafood. Smoked cod and salmon and frozen fish without crumbs are also excellent options.

Couple your fish entrée with tasty vegetables such as spinach, sweet potato chips, green beans or corn, and you've got a flavorful, filing meal.

Now that you know how bene-fish-al these swimmers of the sea are, so go fish!

More Legumes, Please

Hey, leggo my legume. Maybe you aren't sure exactly what a legume is, but you have some vague idea it's part of the vegetable family. Great job! But let's take a closer look at legumes, because they have great taste as well as health benefits for women with PCOS.

Legumes include members of the bean family, such as kidney beans, lima beans, chickpeas, black-eyed peas, lentils, and more. You may have heard the children's rhyme: beans, beans, the musical fruit, the more you eat, the more you toot.

Well, legumes may have a black eye for sometimes causing intestinal gas, but they are not a fruit and not all of them will cause you to pass gas. You can avoid making funny smells by cooking legumes thoroughly in fresh water, rinsing the canned legumes, and eating them on a regular basis. Essentially, your body will get more used to digesting them.

Legumes, often considered a superfood, are high in fiber, protein, folate, Vitamin B, and Vitamin C.

If you've been diagnosed with PCOS, then you need food with a low glycemic index, meaning your blood sugar won't spike after you gulp it down, and you want it to be low in calories, filling, nutritious and yet still delicious! Legumes fit the bill.

Typically legumes are sold dried, in cans, or in packets. Depending on how much time you have to prepare your food, you may prefer to go with canned. Dried legumes tend to take longer to prepare, as they require soaking and cooking. Both dried and canned legumes have a long shelf-life, so you can plan to include them in future meals.

How to prepare them? You can use legumes in soups, such as minestrone or lentil. Create your own version of a veggie burger with chickpeas. Make hummus from chickpeas, and serve it on a platter with warm pita bread. Southwestern-style salads with corn and black beans are often family favorites. Red beans and rice, made with kidney beans, can warm a stomach on a cold winter day. If you're in the mood for Asian, try mixing in almonds or green soy beans into your stir-fry dish.

No matter which type of legume you prefer, including them in your diet can help you fight the symptoms of PCOS by eating food with a low glycemic index. You'll be filled and enjoy the benefits of the additional vitamins and minerals.

Go Nuts for Nuts

Go nuts for nuts if you've got PCOS! You can have a shell of a great diet by including nuts in your meals and snacks on a regular basis.

I THOUGHT NUTS WERE FATTENING?

No way! Nuts are excellent sources of important vitamins and minerals. Eating nuts in the right portions can reduce your risk of heart disease and Type 2 diabetes. As someone with PCOS, you are at a greater risk for diabetes, so nuts can only help! Additionally, snacking on nuts can curb your appetite, so you are less likely to overeat when mealtime comes around.

ARE YOU SURE?

Still not convinced? Well, get this: nuts have very little saturated fat, they contain mass amounts of fiber, they include Vitamin E, folate, copper, magnesium, and even omega-3 fats. In a nutshell, they are packed with powerful health benefits.

WHICH KINDS OF NUTS ARE ESPECIALLY GOOD FOR ME?

Consider walnuts and pecans. These have high levels of omega-3 fats. They can be used in a variety of ways, such as on salads and in cereals, breads, and desserts. Other tasty types include hazelnuts, almonds, sunflower seeds, pumpkin seeds, linseeds, sesame seeds, pine nuts, cashews and macadamia nuts. Crack open some new kinds, and you'll see how each flavor differs from nut to nut.

ENOUGH PUNS FROM THE PEANUT GALLERY.

Peanuts are excellent sources of minerals and nutrients such as niacin, folate, fiber and protein. Their monounsaturated fat works against heart disease. However, peanuts are not actually nuts! They are legumes, in the bean family. Still good for you, though, with their ample supply of manganese, protein, Vitamin B3…the list goes on.

HOW CAN I INCLUDE NUTS IN MY MEALS?

You can try spreading them on your toast or crackers in the form of butter. Many grocery stores carry almond butter, cashew butter, and of course, peanut butter!

You can sprinkle them over your salad for a nutty flavor. Toss them into your cake or muffin mixes. Or grind them up and include them in your own homemade pesto sauce. Many people eat them raw as a snack – but keep yourself under 30 grams per day.

Conclusion

PCOS, or Polycystic Ovarian Syndrome, is a difficult diagnosis but does not have to control your life. By using natural remedies, you can manage your symptoms and lower your risk of also getting diabetes or having a heart attack.

The insulin resistance of PCOS results in a hormonal imbalance and high levels of both insulin and glucose in the blood stream. The symptoms of PCOS usually include, but are not limited to, insulin resistance, ovarian cysts, acne, lack of ovulation or periods, infertility, scalp hair loss, and male-patterned hair growth or hirsutism. Although there is no known cure yet for PCOS, these symptoms can be alleviated by improving your diet and exercise habits or taking other steps to improve your body's sensitivity to insulin.

Here's a recap of the practical steps you can take:

Exercise regularly.

Aim to keep your weight at the right ratio with your height. Plan to make 4-6 cardio workouts of 45 minutes each part of your routine for permanent weight loss. When you are exercising, monitor your heart rate to ensure it is in your target heart rate. If you aren't usually active, start small by taking stairs instead of the elevator, take walks with friends or neighbors, and find opportunities to get moving!

Plan and stick to a healthy diet.

A healthy diet and nutrition is important for everyone, but as someone with PCOS, selecting foods with a low glycemic index is especially important. Look for lean meats, lowfat dairy products, plenty of fruits, legumes, and vegetables, and nuts. Plan small meals with proper portion sizes throughout your day so that you avoid binge-eating. Regularly include supplements such as cinnamon, which will help you increase your body's sensitivity to insulin.

Ask for emotional support.

PCOS isn't easy, and the emotional effects of your diagnosis can be overwhelming. It's normal and natural to feel angry, frustrated, or depressed. Remember you aren't alone – over 10% of women in the U.S. also have PCOS.

Develop a support group of those who you know love you and want the best for you. Ask them to hold you accountable to your goals for weight loss and nutrition. Include your doctor in your support group. Find out if other women in your area are working through PCOS, or search online for a local support group. Let your church group, friend network or others know the general symptoms and reasons for what you are going through so they can support you more effectively.

Your new identity

PCOS isn't who you are, but it is part of your identity. Continue learning about its effects by talking with your doctor and searching for the answers to your questions on reliable, professional sources. The more you understand the effects of PCOS on your body, the more you'll be able to regain control of your health.

RESOURCES

"Acanthosis nigricans." U.S. National Library of Medicine. PubMed Health. http://www.ncbi.nlm.nih.gov/pubmedhealth/PMH0001855/

ANDROGEN EXCESS DISORDERS IN WOMEN: POLYCYSTIC OVARY SYNDROME AND OTHER DISORDERS. Second Edition. Contemporary Endocrinology. Ed. Ricardo Azziz, John E. Nestler, Didier Diwailly. Humana Press. Totowa, New Jersey: 2006. Accessed 3-6-12.

http://www.scribd.com/doc/36327773/Androgen-Excess-Disorders-in-Women#outer_page_161

"Cinnamon for PCOS Weight Loss." eHow.com. Accessed 3-5-12. http://www.ehow.com/way_5647803_cinnamon-pcos-weight-loss.html#ixzz1oIgjoxOW

"Following a Cardio Plan for Weight Loss." Dummies.com.

Accessed 3-13-12. http://www.dummies.com/how-to/content/following-a-cardio-plan-for-weight-loss.html?cid=embedlink

Hairfacts.com. Accessed 3-6-12. www.hairfacts.com.

"How to Stop Hair Loss with PCOS." eHow.com. Accessed 3-6-12. http://www.ehow.com/how_5603015_stop-hair-loss-pcos.html#ixzz1oIcgIlwB

"Jillian Michaels Biography." A+E Television Networks, LLC. Accessed 3-6-2012. http://www.biography.com/people/jillian-michaels-5948?page=2

"Polycystic ovary syndrome fact sheet." Womenshealth.gov. Accessed 3-9-12. http://www.womenshealth.gov/publications/our-publications/fact-sheet/polycystic-ovary-syndrome.cfm

Sherwood, Chris. "How Can I Thicken My Hair Naturally?" Livestrong.com. 5-5-2011. Accessed 3-5-12. http://www.livestrong.com/article/69894-can-thicken-hair-naturally/#ixzz1oOkPyTbS

"The Hormones: Androgens." Tulane/Xavier Center for Bioenvironmental Research. Accessed 3-6-12.

http://e.hormone.tulane.edu/learning/androgens.html

THE NEW GLUCOSE REVOLUTION GUIDE TO LIVING WELL WITH PCOS. Dr. Jennie Brand-Miller, Dr. Nadir R. Farid, Kate Marsh. Da Capo Press: Philadelphia, 2004.

"Your Target Heart Rate." TheWalkingSite.com. Accessed 3-13-12. http://www.thewalkingsite.com/thr.html

http://clinicaltrials.gov/ct2/show/NCT01483118 (potential contacts on Columbia University study)

http://www.fatsoff.com/diseases-related-to-obesity/61-cinnamon-benefits-for-pcos.html

http://women.webmd.com/tc/polycystic-ovary-syndrome-pcos-symptoms

http://pcos.insulitelabs.com/PCOS-Frequently-Asked-Questions.php#PCOS%20Symptoms

http://www.somaacupuncture.com/PCOS.html -- San Francisco Natural Medicine

http://www.ovarian-cysts-pcos.com/supplements.html

http://www.natural-hormone-health.com/natural-treatments-for-PCOS.html

http://www.pcosnomore.com/

http://pcosinfo.com/herbal-remedies-and-pcos/

http://www.polycystic-ovary-syndrome-guide.com/natural-cures.html

http://www.medicinenet.com/skin_tag/article.htm

http://pcosdiva.com/

Exclusive Bonus Download: Gluten Free Living Secrets

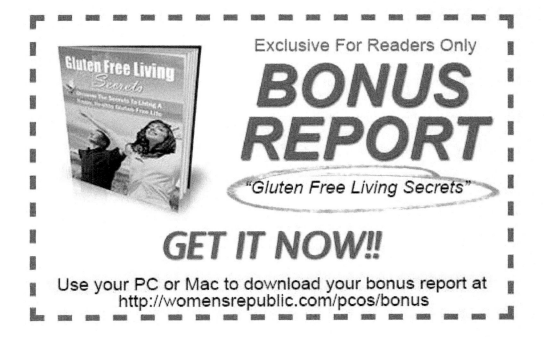

Download your bonus, please visit the download link above from your PC or MAC. To open PDF files, visit http://get.adobe.com/reader/ to download the reader if it's not already installed on your PC or Mac. To open ZIP files, you may need to download WinZip from http://www.winzip.com. This download is for PC or Mac ONLY and might not be downloadable to kindle.

Are you sick and tired of trying every weight loss program out there and failing to see results? Or are you frustrated with not feeling as energetic as you used to despite what you eat? Perhaps you always seem to have a bit of a " dodgy stomach " and indigestion seems to be a regular part of your life?

There's nothing worse than sitting down to a nice big plate of pasta and enjoying your meal only to be met with a growling stomach and the inevitable rush to the toilet.

It's that bloated feeling you get after eating a piece of bread that just " doesn't seem right " . Almost as if you've eaten something poisonous.

Gluten Free Living Secrets is a complete resource that will tell you everything you need to know about the dangers of eating gluten and how to go about transitioning yourself and your family to a life free of this dangerous substance.

Here's just a taste of what you will discover inside Gluten Free Living Secrets:

- What foods you should focus on when first switching to a gluten-free diet

- The 9 grains that are safe and gluten-free

- The truth about whether you can eat pasta on a gluten-free diet

- What you should know to determine if you have Celiac Disease

- and that's not all...

- Why you may want to consider eliminating gluten from your child's diet

- The top 10 reasons to go gluten-free

- How to transform your pantry to be gluten-free

- A list of essential gluten-free shopping tips

- How to keep your kids happy around their gluten-eating friends

- Tips on staying gluten-free when eating out

Gluten Free Living Secrets comes in a digital PDF format that is easy to read either on your computer or on your eBook reader.

Visit the URL above to download this guide and start achieving your overall health and weight loss goals NOW

One Last Thing...

Thank you so much for reading my book. I hope you really liked it. As you probably know, many people look at the reviews on Amazon before they decide to purchase a book. If you liked the book, could you please take a minute to leave a review with your feedback? 60 seconds is all I'm asking for, and it would mean the world to me.

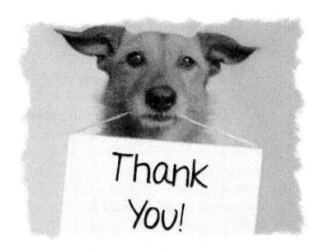

******

Books by This Author:

Permanently Beat Bacterial Vaginosis

Permanently Beat Yeast Infection & Candida

Permanently Beat Urinary Tract Infections

Permanently Beat Hypothyroidism Naturally

Permanently Beat PCOS

The Permanently Beat PCOS Diet & Exercise Shortcuts

The Permanently Beat Hypothyroidism Diet & Exercise Shortcuts

About the Author

Caroline D. Greene is a mother of 2 wonderful girls and a wife to a supportive husband. She has dedicated the past seven years to researching the various women's health topics that are not being openly discussed and providing help and support to the women dealing with these issues in their daily life.

Caroline D. Greene

Published by Women's Republic

Atlanta, Georgia USA

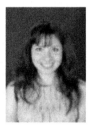

CPSIA information can be obtained
at www.ICGtesting.com
Printed in the USA
LVOW04s2150030717
540265LV00005B/316/P

9 781483 967905